MCQs for the MRCPsych Part II

by
Dr Michael I. Levi, MB, BS(Lond.), MRCPsych Part I
Senior House Officer in Psychiatry,
The London Hospital Rotational Training Scheme,
London, UK

with a Foreword by
Dr Michael A. Reveley, MD, MRCPsych
Senior Lecturer and Consultant in Psychiatry,
The London Hospital Medical College

KLUWER ACADEMIC PUBLISHERS

DORDRECHT - BOSTON - LONDON

Distributors

for the United States and Canada: Kluwer Academic Publishers, PO Box 358, Accord Station, Hingham, MA 02018-0358, USA
for all other countries: Kluwer Academic Publishers Group, Distribution Center, PO Box 322, 3300 AH Dordrecht, The Netherlands

British Library Cataloguing in Publication Data

Levi, Michael I., *1960 –*
 MCQs for the MRCPsych part II.
 1. Medicine. Psychiatry – Questions & answers
 I. Title
 616.89'0076

 ISBN 0-7462-0093-5

Library of Congress Cataloging in Publication Data

Levi, Michael I., 1960 –
 MCQs for the MRCPsych part II.

 Bibliography: p.
 1. Psychiatry – Examinations, questions, etc.
 I. Title. [DNLM: 1. Psychiatry – examination questions.
 WM 18 L664ma]
 RC457.L483   1988   616.89'0076   88-8841
 ISBN 0-7462-0093-5 (pbk.)

Copyright

Published in the United Kingdom by Kluwer Academic Publishers, PO Box 55, Lancaster, UK.

Kluwer Academic Publishers BV incorporates the publishing programmes of D. Reidel, Martinus Nijhoff, Dr W. Junk and MTP Press.

Printed in Great Britain by Butler and Tanner, Frome and London

Contents

Foreword

The examination process is a topic of interest to both trainees and examiners alike. Ideally, examinations should offer the well trained clinician an opportunity to demonstrate his skills and should screen out those who do not reach an acceptable standard. Unfortunately, the examination process itself may get in the way, so that some qualified candidates do not pass simply because they are not 'exam wise'. It is in this regard that Dr Levi's book will be especially helpful. It is not, of course, a substitute for extensive clinical experience and training or a wide reading in psychiatry. It will, however, provide trainees with an opportunity to test their knowledge in a format identical to the new MCQ examination. In this way it will serve as a very useful adjunct to those preparing for the new membership examination.

Dr Michael A. Reveley
Senior Lecturer and Consultant in Psychiatry,
The London Hospital Medical College,
London, UK

Introduction

As from May 1988, the membership examination for the MRCPsych is changing its format considerably. It will consist of two MCQ papers – one covering basic sciences, the other covering clinical topics. Each paper will consist of 50 questions to be completed in 90 minutes. In addition, there will be a traditional essay question paper, a short answer question paper, a clinical examination and a patient management problem oral examination.

In the traditional essay question paper, the candidate has to choose one question out of six, all of which are 'integrated' in the sense of having both basic science and clinical aspects. The time allowed is 90 minutes.

In the short answer question paper, the candidate has to answer 20 compulsory questions. Equal emphasis will be placed on basic sciences and clinical topics i.e. there will be the same number of questions under each of these headings; this may necessitate the use of integrated questions. The time allowed is 90 minutes.

This is to be contrasted with the previous format of the membership examination – this consisted of one MCQ paper of 60 questions to be completed in two hours, a traditional essay question paper, a clinical examination and an oral examination.

The old format of the membership examination tested the candidate on purely clinical topics in psychiatry. This is in marked contrast with the new format of the examination, which tests the candidate equally on both basic sciences and clinical topics. The new examination will be known as the MRCPsych Part II.

The membership examination of the MRCPsych will run concurrently with the MRCPsych Part II from May 1988 to May 1992. Thereafter, only the MRCPsych Part II will be set.

The purpose of writing this book is to give candidates for the MRCPsych Part II adequate practice at the types of MCQs they will encounter. I have restricted my questions to prepare the candidate for the MCQ paper on clinical topics (may I refer candidates to my first book[1] for practice on MCQs in basic sciences). In this way, candidates for the membership examination of the MRCPsych will also find the book helpful.

I have based my questions on the relevant chapters of what is generally regarded to be the most useful textbook[2] to prepare for the MRCPsych Part II examination, with respect to the clinical topics. Candidates will benefit most from reading a particular chapter of this book, and then seeing if they can answer the appropriate section of MCQs. If they then re-read the same chapter, they will hopefully find that my questions will help to re-inforce the more important points in the chapter.

The distribution of questions set on each chapter is based on the sample MCQ paper (clinical topics) issued by the Royal College of Psychiatrists.

References

1. Levi, M.I. (1987). *MCQs for the MRCPsych Part I.* (Lancaster: MTP Press)
2. Gelder, M., Gath, D., Mayou, R. (1986). *Oxford Textbook of Psychiatry.* (Oxford: Oxford Medical Publications)

Acknowledgements

I wish to thank Dr Michael Reveley for providing a Foreword to this book. A special thankyou must go to Mr A.D. Morris of E. Merck Ltd. who helped me to secure the publication of my material.

Thanks once again to Dr J.M. Brewis of MTP Press for giving me the opportunity to publish this sequel to my first book. A final thankyou to my parents for their encouragement and support while producing the book.

Examination Technique

The MCQ paper consists of 50 stems with 5 responses to each stem. The candidate must answer 'true' or 'false' to each response. The following marking scheme is in operation:

> A correctly answered response scores +1
> An incorrectly answered response scores −1
> An unanswered response scores 0

There is a maximum score of 250 marks available. To pass the examination, a mark of between 55–60% will be required i.e. the candidate must achieve a nett score of 138–150 marks out of 250 marks.

Following the advice given in my first book to answer all the responses, candidates might find it useful to know that the number of 'true' responses to stems roughly follows a normal distribution i.e. the 50 stems in the exam can be broken down according to the number of 'true' responses:

Number of 'true' responses	Number of stems	
0	3	(6%)
1	7	(14%)
2	15	(30%)
3	15	(30%)
4	7	(14%)
5	3	(6%)

Total   50

Thus, 60% of the 50 stems can be expected to have 2 or 3 'true' responses, while only 12% of the stems can be expected to have 0 or 5 'true' responses.

This information is helpful when it comes to making educated guesses. For example, consider the question:

Variations of hysteria include

A.   susto
B.   amok
C.   windigo
D.   latah
E.   koro

You may know that responses B and D are true and that response C is false. You may also think that responses A and E are also true, but you are not sure.

Knowing that there is a 60% chance of any given stem having 2 or 3 'true' responses, you should mark responses B and D as 'true', while marking responses A, C and E as 'false'.

Even if one of the responses A or E turns out to be true, you would still end up with a nett score of 3/5 or 60% on this question.

In fact, both responses A and E are false, so you would score 5/5 or 100% on the question!

Personality Disorder

1.   The following associations are correct

A.   Prichard and psychopathic inferiority
B.   Koch and moral insanity
C.   Pinel and *manie sans delire*
D.   Kraeplin and psychopathic personality
E.   Schneider and psychopathic states

2.   The ICD 9 classification includes

A.   asthenic
B.   schizotypal
C.   narcissistic
D.   passive dependent
E.   anankastic

3.   The DSM III classification includes

A.   hysterical
B.   affective
C.   paranoid
D.   schizoid
E.   borderline

4.   Features of obsessional personality disorder include

A.   enjoyment of receiving gifts
B.   indecision
C.   humour
D.   insensitivity to criticism
E.   moralistic in opinions

5.   Features of histrionic personality disorder include

A.   sexual provocation with frigidity
B.   egocentricity
C.   sustained enthusiasms
D.   self-deception
E.   consideration for others

6. **Features of paranoid personality disorder include**

A. argumentative
B. self-importance
C. making friendships easily
D. self-sufficient
E. devious

7. **Features of affective personality disorder include**

A. hypomania
B. endogenous depression
C. subgroup of cycloid personality disorder
D. psychotic depression
E. subgroup of hyperthymic personality disorder

8. **Features of schizoid personality disorder include**

A. extensive inner fantasy world
B. several intimate friendships
C. self-sufficient
D. introspective
E. callous

9. **Features of antisocial personality disorder include**

A. learn from adverse experiences
B. make loving relationships
C. guilt
D. stable work record
E. superficial charm

10. **Features of explosive personality disorder include**

A. several difficulties in relationships
B. generally prone to antisocial behaviour
C. stability of mood with outbursts of anger
D. outbursts readily controllable by individual
E. outbursts invariably confined to words

11. **Features of asthenic personality disorder include**

A.   vigour
B.   responsibility
C.   self-reliance
D.   also called passive personality disorder
E.   also called dependent personality disorder

12. **Features of schizotypal personality disorder include**

A.   interest in telepathy
B.   odd forms of speech
C.   superstitious ideas
D.   unrealistic thinking
E.   interest in clairvoyance

13. **Narcissistic personality disorder frequently overlaps with**

A.   paranoid personality disorder
B.   schizoid personality disorder
C.   borderline personality disorder
D.   histrionic personality disorder
E.   antisocial personality disorder

14. **Features of avoidant personality disorder include**

A.   emotionally cold
B.   high self-esteem
C.   detached from other people
D.   shy
E.   hypersensitive to rejection

15. **Features of borderline personality disorder include**

A.   chronic anhedonia
B.   brief psychotic episodes
C.   superficially socially adapted
D.   identity confusion
E.   stable intense relationships

16.   Features of passive – aggressive personality disorder include

A.   stubbornness
B.   pretended forgetfulness
C.   procrastination
D.   deliberate inefficiency
E.   dawdling

17.   Sjobring's classification for personality includes

A.   reliability
B.   validity
C.   capacity
D.   solidity
E.   stability

18.   Kretschmer's body build types include

A.   ectomorphy
B.   viscerotonia
C.   mesomorphy
D.   somatotonia
E.   endomorphy

19.   Causes of antisocial personality disorder may include

A.   failure of social learning
B.   behaviour disorders in childhood
C.   separation of young child from mother
D.   delay in cerebral maturation
E.   chromosomal abnormalities

20.   Treatment of antisocial personality disorder includes

A.   anxiolytic drugs for short periods
B.   the therapeutic community
C.   small group therapy
D.   individual psychotherapy
E.   major tranquillizers for long periods

Neurosis

1. **Features of anxiety neurosis include**

A.   sensitivity to noise
B.   furrowed brow
C.   borborygmi
D.   difficulty in expiration
E.   decreased frequency of micturition

2. **Other features of anxiety neurosis include**

A.   amenorrhoea
B.   rotational dizziness
C.   early morning wakening commonly
D.   tinnitus
E.   'night terrors'

3. **Neurocirculatory asthenia is also known as**

A.   irritable neuropathy
B.   effort syndrome
C.   Da Costa's syndrome
D.   irritable heart
E.   asthenic syndrome

4. **Differential diagnosis of anxiety neurosis includes**

A.   phaeochromocytoma
B.   hyperglycaemia
C.   alcohol dependence
D.   presenile dementia
E.   schizophrenia

5. **Treatment of anxiety neurosis includes**

A.   psychosurgery
B.   tricyclic antidepressants
C.   benzodiazepines
D.   relaxation training
E.   monoamine oxidase inhibitors

6.   **Simple phobic neuroses include**

A.   acrophobia
B.   agoraphobia
C.   social phobia
D.   illness phobia
E.   arachnophobia

7.   **Differential diagnosis of agoraphobia usually includes**

A.   schizophrenia
B.   senile dementia
C.   paranoid state
D.   hypomania
E.   depression

8.   **Features of social phobic neurosis include**

A.   persecutory feelings
B.   obsessions
C.   nausea
D.   depersonalization
E.   depression

9.   **Themes for other phobic neuroses include**

A.   dental treatment
B.   vomiting
C.   space phobia
D.   excretion
E.   flying

10.   **Treatment of phobic neuroses includes**

A.   implosion
B.   modelling
C.   anxiolytic drugs
D.   antipsychotic drugs
E.   antidepressant drugs

11.   Features of obsessional neuroses include

A.   obsessional quickness
B.   obsessional images
C.   depersonalization
D.   anxiety
E.   thought insertion

12.   Differential diagnosis of obsessional neuroses usually includes

A.   paranoid state
B.   organic cerebral disorders
C.   schizophrenia
D.   mania
E.   drug dependence

13.   Obsessional neuroses definitely improve with

A.   'thought stopping'
B.   clomipramine
C.   psychoanalytic psychotherapy
D.   leucotomy
E.   supportive psychotherapy

14.   Features of hysterical dissociation include

A.   pseudocyesis
B.   aphonia
C.   anaesthesia
D.   mutism
E.   globus hystericus

15.   Features of hysterical conversion include

A.   somnabulism
B.   fugue
C.   multiple personality
D.   hysterical pseudodementia
E.   psychogenic amnesia

16. Features of the Ganser syndrome include

A. hysterical dissociation symptoms
B. malingering
C. 'approximate answers'
D. hysterical conversion symptoms
E. pseudohallucinations

17. Features of hysterical seizures include

A. unconsciousness
B. cyanosis
C. incontinence
D. normal EEG findings
E. bitten tongue

18. Features of epidemic hysteria include

A. only occurs in women
B. typically starts in several people
C. dizziness
D. not seen in schoolchildren
E. 'dancing manias' of the Middle Ages

19. Features of Briquet's syndrome include

A. onset before age 35
B. always female
C. coined by St Pancras Group
D. organic basis rarely present
E. multiple physical symptoms

20. Variations of hysteria include

A. susto
B. amok
C. windigo
D. latah
E. koro

21. **Differential diagnosis of hysteria usually includes**

A. partial complex seizures
B. malingering
C. histrionic personality
D. schizophrenia
E. paranoid state

22. **Features of the Munchausen syndrome include**

A. described by Asher in 1955
B. more common in women
C. also called 'illness addiction' syndrome
D. conscious simulation of symptoms
E. deception of medical staff

23. **Treatment of hysteria characteristically includes**

A. specific methods of behaviour therapy
B. long-term exploratory psychotherapy
C. abreaction
D. medication
E. reassurance

24. **Features of depersonalization neurosis include**

A. dulled emotions
B. mechanical actions
C. déjà vu
D. more common in men
E. insidious onset

25. **Differential diagnosis of depersonalization neurosis includes**

A. hysteria
B. schizoid personality disorder
C. schizophrenia
D. temporal lobe epilepsy
E. obsessional neurosis

26. Treatment of primary depersonalization neurosis usually includes

A. behaviour treatment
B. short trial of an anxiolytic drug
C. short trial of an antipsychotic drug
D. exploratory psychotherapy
E. encouragement to tolerate symptoms

27. Characteristic features of hypochondriasis include

A. pain in 90% of patients
B. biliousness
C. body odours
D. bad taste in mouth
E. right-sided chest pain

28. The most frequent primary disorders in hypochondriasis are

A. anxiety states
B. schizophrenia
C. hysteria
D. dementia
E. depression

29. Hypochondriasis is more common in

A. women
B. elderly
C. higher social classes
D. non-european cultures when secondary to depression
E. those closely associated with disease

30. Effective treatment of primary hypochondriasis includes

A. discussion of the symptoms
B. behaviour therapy
C. anxiolytic drugs
D. supportive measures
E. leucotomy in intractable cases

Affective Disorders

1.   Features of moderate depressive disorder include

A.   reduced rate of blinking
B.   a smiling exterior
C.   irritability
D.   lethargy
E.   diarrhoea

2.   Other features of moderate depressive disorder include

A.   delay in falling asleep
B.   increased appetite
C.   weight gain
D.   'depressive cognitions'
E.   hypochondriacal preoccupations

3.   Features of severe depressive disorder include

A.   also called neurotic depression
B.   auditory hallucinations
C.   visual hallucinations
D.   persecutory delusions
E.   pseudohallucinations

4.   Features of Cotard's syndrome include

A.   nihilistic ideas
B.   more common in men
C.   mutism
D.   rarely associated with irritability
E.   hallucinations

5.   Features of agitated depression include

A.   commoner in younger patients
B.   regarded as a mixed affective state
C.   increased thought tempo
D.   underactivity
E.   also called excited depression

6. **Features of depressive stupor include**

A. echolalia
B. periods of excitement
C. echopraxia
D. mutism
E. motor retardation

7. **Features of mild depressive disorder include**

A. hysterical symptoms
B. early morning wakening
C. hallucinations
D. obsessional symptoms
E. phobias

8. **Features of mania include**

A. diurnal rhythm of mood
B. insomnia with fatigue
C. good appetite with weight gain
D. anger
E. transient depression

9. **Mixed affective states include**

A. depressive stupor
B. manic stupor
C. excited mania
D. unproductive depression
E. inhibited depression

10. **Features of manic stupor include**

A. decreased thought tempo
B. motor acceleration
C. depression
D. described by Kraepelin in 1907
E. fairly commonly seen

11. **Features of typical grief include**

A. excessive guilt
B. blunted emotions
C. anorexia
D. neurosis
E. denial

12. **Classification of depressive disorders by symptom clusters includes**

A. neurotic depressives
B. angry depressives
C. friendly depressives
D. older depressives
E. endogenous depressives

13. **Classification of affective disorders in ICD 9 include**

A. cyclothymic disorder
B. dysthymic disorder
C. affective psychosis
D. atypical affective disorders
E. major affective disorder

14. **Classification of affective disorders in DSM III include**

A. bipolar disorders
B. neurotic depression
C. major depression
D. depressive psychosis
E. unipolar depressive disorder

15. **Differential diagnosis of depressive disorders includes**

A. schizophrenia
B. manic disorders
C. neuroses
D. organic brain syndromes
E. normal sadness

16. Differential diagnosis of manic disorders includes

A. frontal lobe tumour
B. amphetamine abuse
C. schizophrenia
D. depressive disorders
E. general paralysis of the insane

17. Epidemiology of affective disorders includes

A. greater incidence in social class V
B. higher rates in married people
C. autumn and winter peaks for suicide and mania
D. prevalence at 1–2% of general population
E. equal sex prevalence in bipolar disorders

18. 'Depressive spectrum disease' includes

A. antisocial personality disorder
B. hypothyroidism
C. alcoholism
D. general paralysis of the insane
E. iron deficiency anaemia

19. The most relevant personality features predisposing to unipolar depressive disorders include

A. depressive personality disorder
B. schizoid personality disorder
C. readiness to develop anxiety
D. obsessional traits
E. hysterical traits

20. Brown's vulnerability factors in depressive disorder include

A. two or more children under 14 years of age
B. paternal loss before age 11
C. lack of support from husband
D. cyclothymic personality
E. not working outside home

21. **Conditions particularly likely to be followed by depression include**

A. glandular fever
B. taking 'the pill'
C. Parkinsonism
D. disseminated sclerosis
E. influenza

22. **The following associations are correct**

A. Beck and depression conditioned by repeated past losses
B. Seligman and 'maternal deprivation'
C. Freud and loss of love object
D. Wolpe and 'negative cognitive trait'
E. Bowlby and 'learned helplessness'

23. **Correctly linked neurotransmitters and metabolites include**

A. dopamine and HVA
B. adrenaline and MHPG
C. noradrenaline and 5HIAA
D. dopamine and VMA
E. serotonin and 5HT

24. **Endocrine abnormalities in depression include**

A. increased TSH response
B. decreased GH response
C. dexamethasone suppression rarely resisted
D. associated with hypoparathyroidism
E. associated with Addison's disease

25. **Tyrer advocates the use of MAOIs in**

A. phobic and generalised anxiety
B. endogenous depresison
C. some hypochondriacal and obsessional disorders
D. psychotic depression
E. anxiety depressions

26. **Treatment of depressive disorder may include**

A. sleep deprivation
B. vanadium-reducing diet
C. sodium valproate
D. cognitive therapy
E. psychosurgery

27. **Prophylaxis of bipolar affective disorders includes**

A. chlorpromazine
B. carbamazepine
C. lithium
D. haloperidol
E. dothiepin

28. **Treatment of acute mania usually includes**

A. lithium carbonate
B. ECT
C. chlorpromazine
D. haloperidol
E. Valium

29. **Treatments with proven effectiveness in resistant depression include**

A. tri-iodothyronine
B. MAOIs
C. lithium
D. maximising dose of tricyclic antidepressant
E. chlorpromazine

30. **Predictors of a good response to ECT include**

A. hypochondriasis
B. psychotic features
C. hysterical features
D. endogenous features
E. biological features

Schizophrenia

1. **High prevalence of schizophrenia occurs in**

A. Canadian Catholics
B. South-East Jugoslavia
C. Eire
D. Hutterites
E. Southern Sweden

2. **Features of acute schizophrenia include**

A. disorientation
B. Vorbeireden
C. euphoria
D. poverty of thought
E. Mitgehen

3. **Other features of acute schizophrenia include**

A. gustatory hallucinations
B. verbigeration
C. automatic obedience
D. depression
E. impaired memory

4. **Features of chronic schizophrenia include**

A. incontinence
B. suicidal attempts
C. neologisms
D. 'age disorientation'
E. ambitendence

5. **Kraepelin's subtypes of dementia praecox include**

A. paraphrenic
B. complex
C. paranoid
D. catatonic
E. hebephrenic

6. **Bleuler's primary symptoms include**

A. catatonia
B. abnormal behaviours
C. delusions
D. hallucinations
E. blunting of affect

7. **Bleuler's accessory symptoms include**

A. disturbances of associations
B. changes in emotional reactions
C. preference for reality to phantasy
D. ambivalence
E. autism

8. **Schneider's first-rank symptoms include**

A. 'fourth person' auditory hallucinations
B. visual hallucinations
C. delusional idea
D. delusional perception
E. delusional mood

9. **Schneider's second-rank symptoms include**

A. somatic hallucinations
B. secondary delusions
C. catatonic behaviour
D. 'first person' auditory hallucinations
E. 'second person' auditory hallucinations

10. **Leonhard's non-systematic cycloid psychoses include**

A. schizophasia
B. paraphrenias
C. affect-laden paraphrenia
D. hebephrenias
E. catatonias

11. Terms associated with Langfeldt include

A. demence précoce
B. katatonia
C. dementia paranoides
D. reactive schizophrenias
E. process schizophrenia

12. Countries with broader diagnostic criteria for schizophrenia in the IPSS include

A. Taiwan
B. Canada
C. USA
D. USSR
E. India

13. Causes of 'symptomatic schizophrenia' include

A. alcohol abuse
B. encephalitis
C. complex partial seizures
D. a pre-operative syndrome
E. a post-operative syndrome

14. Traditional subgroups of schizophrenia include

A. latent schizophrenia
B. pseudoneurotic schizophrenia
C. simple schizophrenia
D. paranoid schizophrenia
E. hebephrenic schizophrenia

15. Leonhard's bipolar cycloid psychoses include

A. anxiety depression psychosis
B. motility psychosis
C. confusion psychosis
D. futility psychosis
E. manic depressive psychosis

16. **Schizoaffective disorders may be described as**

A. 'schizoaffective'
B. 'cycloid'
C. 'oneirophrenic'
D. 'psychogenic'
E. 'schizophreniform'

17. **Features of** *bouffée délirante* **include**

A. insidious onset
B. delusions
C. perplexity
D. prominent mood disturbance
E. poor immediate prognosis

18. **Differential diagnosis of schizophrenia characteristically includes**

A. personality disorder
B. mental handicap
C. affective disorder
D. neurosis
E. organic syndromes

19. **The following associations are correct**

A. Singer and marital schism
B. Birley and marital skew
C. Bateson and abnormal family communications
D. Lidz and double-bind
E. Leff and life events

20. **Features of Crow's type II schizophrenic syndrome include**

A. good response to neuroleptics
B. good prognosis
C. normal brain ventricular size
D. positive symptoms
E. acute onset

21.   The following associations are correct

A.   concrete thinking and Cameron
B.   over-inclusive thinking and Goldstein
C.   construct theory and Bannister
D.   defective filter and Venables
E.   overarousal and Broadbent

22.   Neurotransmitter disturbances in schizophrenia may include

A.   serotonin underactivity
B.   noradrenaline overactivity
C.   dopamine underactivity
D.   serotonin overactivity
E.   noradrenaline underactivity

23.   Factors predicting a poor prognosis in schizophrenia include

A.   older age at onset
B.   being married
C.   low IQ
D.   low social class
E.   no previous psychiatric history

24.   Factors predicting a good prognosis in schizophrenia include

A.   hebephrenic symptomatology
B.   lack of precipitants
C.   prominent affective symptoms
D.   short episode
E.   sudden onset

25.   Delusions occurring in paranoid syndromes include

A.   persecutory
B.   amorous
C.   grandiose
D.   hypochondriacal
E.   jealous

26.   Behavioural treatment for schizophrenia includes

A.   operant conditioning directed to specific symptoms
B.   intensive family therapy
C.   individual psychotherapy
D.   token economies
E.   social skills training

27.   Psychological tests used in schizophrenia include

A.   thematic apperception test
B.   repertory grid
C.   psychoanalysis
D.   Rorschach inkblot test
E.   object sorting procedures

28.   The epidemiology of schizophrenia includes increased

A.   prevalence of right-handedness
B.   incidence in summer births
C.   prevalence of middle social class
D.   incidence of high birth order if from large family
E.   incidence of perinatal injuries

29.   'Soft' neurological signs in chronic schizophrenia include

A.   dysphasia
B.   astereognosis
C.   clumsiness
D.   gait abnormalities
E.   dysgraphaesthesia

30.   Passivity phenomena include

A.   Wahnstimmung
B.   Gedankenlautwerden
C.   delusions of control
D.   somatic hallucinations
E.   écho de la pensée

Paranoid Symptoms/States

1. **Paranoid symptoms include**

A. ideas of reference
B. delusions of grandiose identity
C. persecutory delusions
D. delusions of grandiose ability
E. delusions of reference

2. **Defence mechanisms causing paranoid symptoms characteristically include**

A. reaction formation
B. sublimation
C. projection
D. displacement
E. denial

3. **Syndromes allied to paranoia include**

A. der sensitive Beziehungswahn
B. Gilles de la Tourette syndrome
C. Cotard's syndrome
D. couvade syndrome
E. sensitive delusions of reference

4. **Primary mental disorders associated with paranoid features characteristically include**

A. personality disorders
B. hebephrenic schizophrenia
C. affective disorders
D. neurosis
E. organic mental states

5. **Features common to both paranoia and paraphrenia include**

A. delusions
B. hallucinations
C. personality deterioration
D. a form of schizophrenia
E. 'late paraphrenia'

6. **The ICD 9 classification of paranoid states includes**

A. paranoia
B. atypical paranoid disorder
C. induced psychosis
D. acute paranoid disorder
E. folie à deux

7. **The DSM III classification of paranoid disorders includes**

A. paranoia
B. shared paranoid disorder
C. paraphrenia
D. psychogenic paranoid psychosis
E. simple paranoid state

8. **Synonyms of pathological jealousy include**

A. psychotic jealousy
B. erotic jealousy
C. sexual jealousy
D. othello syndrome
E. morbid jealousy

9. **Features of pathological jealousy include**

A. overvalued idea in partner's infidelity
B. commoner in women
C. apprehension
D. irritability
E. misery

10. **The most frequent causes of pathological jealousy are**

A. alcoholism
B. depressive illness
C. neurosis and personality disorder
D. paranoid states
E. organic disorders

11.   Synonyms of erotic delusions include

A.   Capgras' syndrome
B.   Ekbom's syndrome
C.   Munro's syndrome
D.   'pure erotomania'
E.   De Clérambault's syndrome

12.   Features of De Clérambault's syndrome include

A.   more common in men
B.   quite commonly seen
C.   supposed lover is usually accessible
D.   described by Enoch and Trethowan in 1959
E.   subject is usually married

13.   Causes of De Clérambault's syndrome include

A.   a 'pure' form of the disease
B.   paranoid schizophrenia
C.   affective disorder
D.   organic mental disturbance
E.   hysterical personality disorder

14.   Themes on which 'reformist delusions' are centred include

A.   medical
B.   political
C.   religious
D.   philosophical
E.   sporting

15.   Features of Capgras' syndrome include

A.   déjà vu
B.   more common in men
C.   derealization
D.   synonymous with 'delusion of doubles'
E.   synonymous with 'illusion of doubles'

16. **Features of the Fregoli syndrome include**

A. originally described by Fregoli
B. usually associated with affective disorders
C. little evidence of an organic aetiological component
D. more common than Capgras' syndrome
E. subject identifies a familiar person in various other people

17. **Features of induced psychosis include**

A. delusions nearly always hypochondriacal
B. more common in men
C. most commonly seen in husband and wife relationship
D. also known as folie du doute
E. all known cases involve members of the same family

18. **Features of monosymptomatic hypochondriacal psychosis include**

A. coenestopathic states
B. hypochondriacal ideas
C. Ekbom's syndrome
D. best treated with sulpiride
E. described by Munro in 1980

19. **Features of sensitive delusions of reference include**

A. exhaustion
B. described by Sheldon
C. personality deterioration
D. conscious minor conflicts
E. also called 'der sensitive Beziehungswahn'

20. **Features of Capgras' syndrome include**

A. part of organic confusion
B. well described by Capgras
C. also called 'l'illusion des sosies'
D. usually part of an affective disorder
E. the misidentified person is often the patient's spouse

Organic Psychiatry

1.   Features of delirium include

A.   clear consciousness
B.   steady, progressive course
C.   insidious onset
D.   'catastrophic reaction'
E.   'organic orderliness'

2.   Features of dementia include

A.   'shrinkage of the milieu'
B.   fluctuating course
C.   impaired consciousness
D.   acute onset
E.   global impairment of cerebral functions

3.   Causes of delirium include

A.   L-DOPA intoxication
B.   exanthemata
C.   alcohol withdrawal
D.   normal pressure hydrocephalus
E.   punch drunk syndrome

4.   Causes of dementia include

A.   cerebral sarcoidosis
B.   post-ictal states
C.   thallium poisoning
D.   digitalis intoxication
E.   subdural haematoma

5.   Features of frontal lobe syndrome include

A.   Witzelsucht
B.   grasp reflex
C.   amnesia
D.   cortical sensory loss
E.   alexia

6. **Features of parietal lobe syndrome include**

A. visual agnosia
B. dysphasia
C. ideational apraxia
D. hemisomatognosia
E. finger agnosia

7. **The main psychiatric causes of stupor include**

A. mania
B. depression
C. hysteria
D. schizophrenia
E. organic causes

8. **Features of Alzheimer's disease include**

A. affects 10% of people over age of 65
B. more common in men
C. decreased risk of Down's syndrome in sufferer's relatives
D. aluminium may be of aetiological significance
E. on average death is within 8 years of diagnosis

9. **Features of Pick's disease include**

A. more common than Alzheimer's disease
B. more common in men
C. cells with argentophile inclusion bodies
D. argentophilic plaques
E. mirror sign

10. **Features of Huntington's chorea include**

A. paranoid psychosis
B. ataxic gait
C. age at onset usually 25 – 50
D. selective loss of 5 HT neurones
E. personality change

11.   Features of Creutzfeld – Jacob disease include

A.   equal sex incidence
B.   parietal signs
C.   myoclonic jerks
D.   psychotic features
E.   flaccidity

12.   Features of normal pressure hydrocephalus include

A.   cranial nerves affected
B.   sensory symptoms in upper limbs
C.   more common in the elderly
D.   slowness
E.   motor symptoms in upper limbs

13.   Psychiatric sequelae of head injury include

A.   'process' schizophrenia
B.   depressive psychosis
C.   hypochondriasis
D.   schizophreniform psychosis
E.   hysterical symptoms

14.   Classic pictures in general paresis include

A.   manic elation
B.   grandiose
C.   neuraesthenic
D.   depressive
E.   paranoid schizophreniform

15.   Features of the punch-drunk syndrome include

A.   paranoid ideation
B.   epilepsy
C.   alcohol intoxication
D.   morbid jealousy
E.   irritability

16. **Features of herpes simplex encephalitis include**

A. apyrexia
B. dementia
C. delirium
D. marked hallucinations
E. insidious onset

17. **Features of multiple sclerosis include**

A. lower motor neurone deficits
B. retrobulbar neuritis
C. also called tuberous sclerosis
D. oculomotor paralysis
E. paraesthesia

18. **Features of systemic lupus erythematosus (SLE) include**

A. steady, progressive mental disturbance
B. chronic organic reaction is commonest
C. cerebral SLE is seen in 90% of cases
D. neurotic reactions are rare
E. schizophreniform psychosis is rare

19. **Features of phaeochromocytoma include**

A. confusion
B. hysteria
C. mania
D. schizophrenia
E. paranoia

20. **Common psychiatric symptoms in acromegaly include**

A. depression
B. delirium
C. agitation
D. lack of initiative
E. apathy

21. **Features of hepatic failure include**

A. specific EEG changes
B. coma
C. irrational behaviour
D. neurological abnormalities
E. insomnia

22. **Features of acute intermittent porphyria include**

A. schizophreniform psychosis
B. delirium
C. depression
D. diarrhoea
E. peripheral neuritis

23. **Features of Wernicke's encephalopathy include**

A. confabulation
B. clear consciousness
C. auditory hallucinations
D. ataxia
E. peripheral neuropathy

24. **Features of subacute combined degeneration of the cord include**

A. anterior column loss
B. negative Shilling test for B_{12} absorption
C. microcytic anaemia
D. lower motor neurone lesions
E. negative pentagastrin test for achlorhydria

25. **Side effects of procyclidine include**

A. drowsiness
B. agitation
C. confusion
D. visual hallucinations
E. disorientation

26. **Features of sodium depletion include**

A. paralytic ileus
B. ECG changes
C. muscle cramps
D. sweating
E. giddiness

27. **Common features of temporal lobe epilepsy include**

A. jamais vu
B. tactile hallucinations
C. automatisms
D. fugues
E. first rank symptoms of schizophrenia

28. **The commonest drugs used to treat petit mal epilepsy include**

A. phenobarbitone
B. carbamazepine
C. sodium valproate
D. primidone
E. ethosuximide

29. **Disorders of initiating and maintaining sleep include**

A. 'restless legs syndrome'
B. sleep apnoea
C. Klein – Levin syndrome
D. jet lag
E. night terrors

30. **Features of narcolepsy include**

A. catalepsy
B. epilepsy
C. insomnia
D. hypnapompic hallucinations
E. schizophrenia-like psychoses

Psychiatry and Medicine

1.   **Organic causes of anxiety include**

A.   hypoventilation
B.   drug withdrawal
C.   hypoglycaemia
D.   phaeochromocytoma
E.   hypothyroidism

2.   **Endocrine abnormalities in anorexia nervosa include**

A.   decreased GH
B.   raised LH
C.   decreased cortisol
D.   raised T_3
E.   raised FSH

3.   **Differential diagnosis of anorexia nervosa includes**

A.   schizophrenia
B.   obsessive/compulsive disorder
C.   reticuloses
D.   hyperpituitarism
E.   myxoedema

4.   **Poor prognostic factors in anorexia nervosa include**

A.   younger age at onset
B.   higher weight during illness
C.   short duration of illness
D.   vomiting
E.   bulimia

5.   **Treatment of anorexia nervosa generally includes**

A.   tricyclic antidepressants
B.   intensive psychoanalytic psychotherapy
C.   behaviour therapy
D.   chlorpromazine
E.   supportive psychotherapy

6. **Features of bulimia nervosa include**

A. renal damage
B. pitted teeth
C. parotid swelling
D. epileptic fits
E. acute dilatation of stomach

7. **Differential diagnosis of bulimia nervosa includes**

A. psychogenic vomiting
B. phobic states
C. hyperthalamic tumours
D. Kleine – Levin syndrome
E. alcohol dependence

8. **Features of the type B behaviour pattern include**

A. ambitiousness
B. preoccupation with deadlines
C. hostility
D. excessive competitive drive
E. chronic sense of urgency

9. **Features of uraemia include**

A. steady, progressive course
B. acute delirium in 75%
C. frequently functional psychosis
D. seizures in 75%
E. depression

10. **Features of tardive dyskinesia include**

A. tics
B. chorea
C. orolingual dyskinesia
D. dystonia
E. athetosis

11. Generally effective remedies for tardive dyskinesia include

A. reserpine
B. benzhexol
C. diazepam
D. tetrabenazine
E. stopping the antipsychotic medication

12. Occupational cramp occurs in

A. telegraphists
B. pianists
C. typists
D. violinists
E. psychiatrists

13. Features of Gilles de la Tourette syndrome include

A. more common in women
B. onset in middle age
C. coprophagia
D. echopraxia
E. echolalia

14. Features of trichotillomania include

A. more common in men
B. usually pubic hair is pulled out
C. intestinal obstruction
D. usually begins in adolescence
E. hairs removed in tufts or individually

15. Features of pseudocyesis include

A. part of hysterical dissociation
B. hyperemesis gravidarum
C. stillbirth
D. amenorrhoea
E. abdominal distention

16.   **Features of the couvade syndrome include**

A.   toothache
B.   morning sickness
C.   nihilistic delusions
D.   approximate answers
E.   surrogate motherhood

17.   **Features of maternity blues include**

A.   impaired cognitive function
B.   more frequent among multigravidae
C.   related to the use of anaesthesia
D.   history of premenstrual tension likely
E.   lability of mood

18.   **Other features of maternity blues include**

A.   increased thirst
B.   sudden weight loss
C.   decreased urinary sodium secretion
D.   symptoms peak on 3rd or 4th postpartum day
E.   unrelated to complications at time of delivery

19.   **Clinical pictures observed in puerperal psychosis include**

A.   paranoid psychosis
B.   affective psychosis
C.   psychogenic psychosis
D.   schizophrenia
E.   acute organic psychosis

20.   **Poor prognosis in puerperal psychosis is indicated by**

A.   an affective psychosis
B.   a positive family psychiatric history
C.   schizophrenia
D.   presence of severe marital problems
E.   neurotic personality

21.   Features of puerperal depression include

A.   affects 30% of women in postpartum period
B.   onset usually within 3 days of delivery
C.   depressive mood is always more prominent than anxiety
D.   less common than puerperal psychosis
E.   less common than maternity blues

22.   Important aetiological factors in puerperal depression include

A.   hormonal effect on tyrosine metabolism
B.   older age
C.   recent stressful events
D.   previous psychiatric history
E.   late postpartum blues

23.   Aetiological theories in premenstrual syndrome include

A.   oestrogen deficiency
B.   aldosterone deficiency
C.   raised MAO activity
D.   progesterone excess
E.   lowered prolactin levels

24.   The premenstrual syndrome may be associated with an increase in

A.   suicide
B.   violent crimes
C.   rape
D.   illness behaviour
E.   parasuicide

25.   Features of the menopause include

A.   sweating
B.   vaginal lubrication
C.   depression
D.   dizziness
E.   headaches

26.   Frequent responses to mastectomy include

A.   marital problems
B.   schizophrenic symptoms
C.   affective symptoms
D.   high self-esteem
E.   sexual problems

27.   Sterilization in women worsens their

A.   mental state
B.   ability to conceive
C.   sexual relationship
D.   social adjustment
E.   general health

28.   The following associations are correct

A.   type B personality and ischaemic heart disease
B.   affection-seeking personality and peptic ulcer
C.   ambitious personality and bronchial asthma
D.   obsessional traits and ulcerative colitis
E.   anxious – histrionic personality and irritable bowel syndrome

29.   The most common psychiatric illnesses provoked by physical illness include

A.   mania
B.   anxiety neuroses
C.   acute organic syndromes
D.   schizophrenia
E.   depressive disorders

30.   The commonest defence mechanisms used by dying patients include

A.   dependency
B.   reaction formation
C.   magic undoing
D.   displacement
E.   denial

Suicide/Deliberate Self-Harm

1.   Suicide rates are higher in

A.   rural than urban areas
B.   adolescent females than adolescent males
C.   the never married than divorcees
D.   December than August
E.   social class III than social class V

2.   Durkheim's main categories of suicide include

A.   egotistic suicide
B.   sedistic suicide
C.   anomic suicide
D.   hedonistic suicide
E.   altruistic suicide

3.   The two most frequent psychiatric causes of suicide include

A.   drug dependency
B.   personality disorder
C.   schizophrenia
D.   alcoholism
E.   depressive disorders

4.   The following associations are correct

A.   attempted suicide and Beck
B.   deliberate self-injury and Catalán
C.   parasuicide and Kessel
D.   non-fatal deliberate self-harm and Kreitman
E.   deliberate self-poisoning and Morgan

5.   Positive correlates of suicide include

A.   redundancy
B.   retirement
C.   immigrant status
D.   family history of alcoholism
E.   separation

6.   **Suicide rates among doctors are highest in**

A.   obstetricians
B.   general surgeons
C.   anaesthetists
D.   general physicians
E.   psychiatrists

7.   **Features of suicide in the 12 – 14-year-old group include**

A.   more common in girls
B.   boys more likely to take drug overdoses
C.   suicidal threats rarely made beforehand
D.   girls more likely to use violent methods
E.   suicidal threats should be investigated

8.   **Features of completed suicide include**

A.   incidence rising
B.   loss of parent by death in early childhood
C.   a precipitant of guilt
D.   often a premeditated setting
E.   usually warning given

9.   **The most commonly used drugs in deliberate self-harm (DSH) include**

A.   antidepressants
B.   barbiturates
C.   major tranquillizers
D.   minor tranquillizers
E.   non-opiate analgesics

10.   **Positive correlates of deliberate self-laceration include**

A.   nursing connections
B.   increased incidence of menstrual irregularity
C.   poor verbalizers
D.   associated bulimia nervosa
E.   increased incidence of hospitalization before age 5

11.   Features of deliberate self-harm include

A.   incidence declining
B.   a broken home in early childhood
C.   major depression in 50% of cases
D.   forewarning always given
E.   poor physical health

12.   Correlates of deliberate self-harm include

A.   higher incidence in middle-class areas
B.   unemployment 15 x expected rate
C.   15 – 20% mentally ill
D.   50% disrupted in interpersonal relationships
E.   previous criminal record in 6% females

13.   Factors predicting suicide after DSH include

A.   drug abuse
B.   female sex
C.   antisocial personality disorder
D.   low social class
E.   previous suicidal attempt

14.   Circumstances suggesting high suicidal intent in DSH include

A.   advance planning
B.   'final acts'
C.   attempts to obtain help afterwards
D.   dangerous method
E.   precautions to avoid discovery

15.   Factors predicting the repetition of DSH include

A.   older age group
B.   criminal record
C.   depressive disorder
D.   social isolation
E.   previous psychiatric treatment

16. **Motives for deliberate self-harm include**

A. relief from state of mind
B. attempt to influence others
C. cry for help
D. escape from intolerable situation
E. 'testing the benevolence of fate'

17. **Symptoms associated with increased suicidal risk include**

A. hypersomnia
B. lack of guilt
C. menopausal symptoms
D. absence of agitation
E. social adequacy

18. **Of the 9% of the general population sample reported feeling suicidal by Paykel (1974)**

A. 1% felt life no longer worthwhile
B. 1% wished themselves dead
C. 3.5% had thought of ending their lives
D. 2.8% seriously contemplated suicide
E. 0.6% actually had made an attempt

19. **Management of deliberate self-laceration generally includes**

A. formal psychotherapy
B. minor tranquillizers
C. major tranquillizers
D. vigorous exercise
E. relaxation techniques

20. **Deliberate self-harm cases may be assessed by**

A. psychiatrists
B. social workers
C. relatives
D. psychiatric nurses
E. junior medical staff

Alcohol/Drug Dependence

1. Features of alcohol dependence syndrome include

A. reinstatement after abstinence
B. decreased tolerance to alcohol
C. stereotyped pattern of drinking
D. repeated withdrawal symptoms
E. prominence of drink-avoiding behaviour

2. Organic sequelae of alcohol dependence include

A. central pontine myelinolysis
B. optic atrophy
C. Marchiafavabignami syndrome
D. cardiomyopathy
E. haemochromatosis

3. Features of fetal alcohol syndrome include

A. psychological under-activity
B. withdrawal symptoms in the neonate
C. cardiovascular defects
D. 17% neonatal mortality
E. limb defects

4. Features of pathological drunkenness include

A. excessive alcohol consumption
B. conspicuous neurological signs of intoxication
C. explosive outbursts of aggression
D. acute psychotic episodes
E. individual idiosyncratic reactions to alcohol

5. Withdrawal symptoms of alcohol dependence include

A. hallucinations
B. hypoacusis
C. sweating (drenching in late evening)
D. euphoric mood disturbance
E. convulsions

6. **Features of delirium tremens include**

A. truncal ataxia
B. hypersomnia
C. hypotension
D. leucopenia
E. symptoms characteristically worse in morning

7. **Features of alcoholic hallucinosis include**

A. clouded consciousness
B. visual hallucinations
C. clear evidence for association with schizophrenia
D. delirium tremens
E. rarely clears in a few days

8. **Excessive drinking is associated with**

A. murder
B. larceny
C. lasting unemployment
D. sexual offences
E. fraud

9. **Epidemiological aspects of excessive drinking include**

A. highest prevalence in 'middle' social classes
B. low prevalence in North American negroes
C. decreased incidence among females
D. low prevalence in urban areas
E. commoner in unmarried than married women

10. **High-risk occupations for alcohol dependence include**

A. psychiatric nurses
B. kitchen porters
C. printers
D. actors
E. doctors

11.   Classic psychoanalytic theory of alcohol dependence includes

A.   anal fixation
B.   oral fixation
C.   overt homosexuality
D.   death-wish
E.   latent homosexuality

12.   Treatment of alcohol withdrawal symptoms includes

A.   chlordiazepoxide
B.   major tranquillizers
C.   minor tranquillizers
D.   tricyclic antidepressants
E.   chlormethiazole

13.   Predictors of good prognosis in alcohol dependence include

A.   ability to defer gratification
B.   younger age
C.   previous treatment
D.   antisocial personality traits
E.   ability to form deep emotional relationships

14.   Deterrents to impulsive drinking include

A.   citrated calcium carbimide
B.   chlorpromazine
C.   lithium
D.   valium
E.   metronidazole

15.   Prevention of alcohol dependence definitely occurs with

A.   mass media propaganda
B.   reducing the price of alcohol
C.   increasing sale restrictions on alcohol
D.   abolishing the advertising of alcohol
E.   classroom lectures

16.   'Controlled' drugs in class B include

A.   benzphetamine
B.   amphetamine
C.   pethidine
D.   mescaline
E.   cannabis

17.   Psychoanalytic theory of drug dependence includes

A.   oral fixation
B.   anal fixation
C.   regression to pregenital anal-erotic level
D.   regression to anal level
E.   regression to oral level

18.   Epidemiological aspects of drug dependence include

A.   incidence falling
B.   slight peak in middle age
C.   more common in women
D.   trend towards single drug misuse
E.   affects all social classes in UK

19.   Opiate withdrawal symptoms include

A.   hypersomnia
B.   constricted pupils
C.   rhinorrhoea
D.   yawning
E.   lacrimation

20.   Clinical features of chronic opiate dependence include

A.   impotence
B.   tremors
C.   dilated pupils
D.   constipation
E.   weakness

21.   Barbiturate withdrawal symptoms include

A.   clear consciousness
B.   hypersomnia
C.   convulsions
D.   hypertension
E.   hallucinations

22.   Clinical features of barbiturate dependence include

A.   nystagmus
B.   dilated pupils
C.   depression
D.   slurred speech
E.   dullness

23.   Features of cannabis dependence include

A.   evidence of teratogenicity
B.   convincing evidence of tolerance
C.   some physical dependence occurs
D.   may lead to a psychosis
E.   a definite withdrawal syndrome

24.   Clinical indications for amphetamines include

A.   appetite supression
B.   narcolepsy
C.   severe depression
D.   hyperkinetic syndrome
E.   obesity

25.   Features of amphetamine psychosis include

A.   tactile hallucinations
B.   persecutory delusions
C.   clouded consciousness
D.   often becomes chronic
E.   auditory hallucinations

26. Features of cocaine dependence include

A. fornication
B. constricted pupils
C. paranoid psychosis
D. depression
E. excitation

27. Features of LSD dependence include

A. 'psychedelic syndrome'
B. schizophreniform psychosis
C. 'flashback' phenomena
D. bradycardia
E. conventional doses associated with chromosomal abnormalities

28. Phencyclidine withdrawal symptoms include

A. euphoria
B. anergia
C. physical discomfort
D. retardation
E. extreme craving

29. Features of solvent abuse include

A. physical dependence common
B. frequent perceptual disturbances
C. sustained and regular abuse in about 50%
D. usually a group activity
E. psychological dependence rare

30. Features of psylocybin dependence include

A. usually smoked
B. physical dependency
C. more intense effects than LSD dependence
D. acute panic
E. 'flashback' phenomena

Psychosexual Problems

1. Classification of sexual problems in ICD 9 includes

A. gender identity disorder of childhood
B. homosexuality
C. bestiality
D. zoophilia
E. ego-dystonic homosexuality

2. Variations of the sexual act include

A. fetishism
B. frotteurism
C. exhibitionism
D. transvestism
E. necrophilia

3. Disorders of sexual arousal include

A. low libido
B. retarded ejaculation
C. dyspareunia
D. transexualism
E. erectile impotence

4. Conditions commonly associated with sexual dysfunction include

A. Addison's disease
B. asthma
C. angina pectoris
D. myxoedema
E. diabetes

5. Drugs that may impair sexual function include

A. probanthine
B. oral contraceptives
C. guanethidine
D. indomethacin
E. benzodiazepines

6.   Positive factors pulling towards homosexuality include

A.   'Peter Pan complex'
B.   failure of heterosexual relationships
C.   lack of confidence in potency
D.   learned inhibition within the family
E.   lack of confidence in masculinity

7.   Features of fetishism include

A.   usually begins in middle age
B.   not described among women
C.   occurs in homosexual men
D.   EEG evidence of temporal lobe dysfunction occasionally
E.   shyness with women

8.   Features of transvestism include

A.   more common in lower social classes
B.   a disorder of core gender identity
C.   may use female clothing for fetishistic masturbation
D.   90% are married
E.   usually evident before age 10

9. Features of paedophilia include:

A.   synonymous with exhibitionism towards young girls
B.   almost invaribaly a disorder of men
C.   10% of children participate actively
D.   95% are relatives or friends of the child
E.   alcohol is rarely involved

10.   Features of exhibitionism include:

A.   victims are usually known
B.   usually occurs in art galleries or museums
C.   commonest single sexual offence
D.   20% only offend once
E.   enjoyment of risk-taking

11. **Features of voyeurism include**

A. occasionally called scopophilia
B. voyeur attempts sexual activity with women
C. most voyeurs reported by passers-by
D. usually associated with masturbation
E. occurs in homosexual men

12. **Features of sexual sadism include**

A. named after Leopold von Sacher
B. 'lust murders'
C. no cases involving animals reported
D. necrophilia
E. behaviour therapy is a proven treatment

13. **Features of sexual masochism include**

A. named after Ladé de Marquis
B. occurs in women
C. unreported in homosexual relationships
D. may be sexual sadism turned inwards
E. satisfactory evidence for treatment by psychoanalysis

14. **Features of transexualism include**

A. not an offence in itself
B. high sex drive
C. usually convinced of 'wrong sex' before age 8
D. disorder of gender role behaviour
E. usually a biological male who is convinced he is a female

15. **The three types of incestuous father characteristically include**

A. ectogamic
B. promiscuous
C. mesogamic
D. paedophilic
E. endogamic

Psychogeriatrics

1. **Features of the normal aging brain include**

A. senile plaques
B. loss of nerve cells
C. thickening of the meninges
D. ischaemic lesions
E. ventricular enlargement

2. **Epidemiology of people aged over 65 includes**

A. constitute 30% of population of Western Europe
B. account for 60% of suicides
C. make up 75% of all long-stay psychiatric patients
D. make up 10% of all psychiatric ward first admissions
E. 15% live alone

3. **Roth's (1955) five diagnostic groups include**

A. senile psychoses
B. anxiety neurosis
C. schizophrenia
D. late paraphrenia
E. chronic confusion

4. **Biochemical changes in senile dementia of the Alzheimer type (SDAT) include**

A. increased acetylcholinesterase
B. increased GABA
C. decreased dopamine-beta-hydroxylase
D. acetylcholine neurone regeneration
E. decreased choline acetyltransferase

5. **Pathological changes in SDAT include**

A. neuritic plaques
B. 'lawless' proliferation of dendritic branches
C. decreased fibrous gliosis
D. granulovacuolar regeneration
E. 'knife-blade' atrophy

6. Clinical features of SDAT include

A. frontal lobe dysfunction
B. parietal lobe dysfunction
C. Parkinsonism
D. usually begins after age of 60
E. euphoric mood

7. Features of benign senescent forgetfulness include

A. progressive syndrome
B. definitely distinct from SDAT
C. difficulty in remembering
D. life expectancy unchanged
E. current status uncertain

8. The aetiology of multi-infarct dementia may include

A. selective reduction in choline acetyltransferase
B. autosomal dominant predisposition
C. a prion-proteinaceous infectious agent
D. selective loss of GABA neurones
E. thromboembolism from extracranial arteries

9. The pathology of multi-infarct dementia includes

A. arteriosclerosis of smaller vessels
B. single micro-infarcts
C. gliosis
D. degree of infarction unrelated to degree of cognitive impairment
E. cystic necrosis

10. Clinical features of multi-infarct dementia include

A. relative preservation of personality
B. 'emotional incontinence'
C. erratic progression
D. insidious onset
E. patchy psychological deficits

11. **Differential diagnosis of dementia includes**

A. schizophrenia
B. depressive disorders
C. Ganser's syndrome
D. paranoid disorders
E. acute organic syndromes

12. **Drugs of specific benefit in SDAT definitely include**

A. hydergine
B. cerebral vasodilators
C. piracetam
D. anticoagulants
E. hyperbaric oxygen

13. **Epidemiology of elderly depressive disorder includes**

A. first, severe disorders are rare between ages 50 and 70
B. elderly suicide is not usually associated with depressive disorder
C. in medical wards, it is rarely unrecognised
D. in general practice, it is rarely unrecognised
E. 20% are referred to psychiatrists within first 6 months of illness

14. **Features of elderly depressive disorder include**

A. agitation
B. severe retardation
C. nihilistic delusions
D. hallucinations of an obscene kind
E. symptoms often more striking than in younger people

15. **Post (1985) subdivided elderly depression into**

A. senile melancholia
B. psychotic depressives
C. hostile depressives
D. anxious depressives
E. younger depressive with personality disorder

16.   Features of depressive pseudodementia include

A.   conspicuous difficulty in concentration
B.   presence of focal signs
C.   impaired memory function on careful clinical testing
D.   relatively acute onset
E.   communication of distress

17.   Differential diagnosis of elderly depressive disorder usually includes

A.   paranoid disorder
B.   schizo-affective disorder
C.   dementia
D.   mania
E.   neurosis

18.   Elderly hypomania is characterised by

A.   infectious gaiety
B.   marked flight of ideas
C.   depressive and manic symptoms combined
D.   frequently recurrent symptoms
E.   higher incidence than hypomania in younger people

19.   Features of late paraphrenia include

A.   relatively poor preservation of personality
B.   more common in married patients
C.   accounts for 20% of first admissions among elderly
D.   more common in females
E.   tends to run a chronic course

20.   Post (1966) divided elderly paranoid conditions into

A.   paranoid hallucinosis
B.   schizophrenia with first rank symptoms
C.   paraphrenia
D.   schizophrenia with paranoid symptoms
E.   late paraphrenia

21.   Differential diagnosis of elderly paranoid states includes

A.   paranoid personality
B.   schizophrenia
C.   neurosis
D.   affective disorders
E.   organic mental disorders

22.   Good prognostic indicators in elderly affective disorder include

A.   ventricular enlargement
B.   senile habitus
C.   organic brain disease
D.   short duration of illness
E.   onset before age of 70

23.   Causal factors in late paraphrenia may include

A.   'social isolation' due to deafness
B.   personality abnormalities
C.   presence of surviving relatives
D.   living alone at onset of illness
E.   organic brain disease

24.   Marked features of apathetic depression include

A.   second person auditory hallucinations
B.   self-neglect
C.   delusions of filth
D.   social withdrawal
E.   loss of interest

25.   Increased prevalence of elderly affective disorder is seen if

A.   past psychiatric history of neurotic disorder
B.   presence of physical health
C.   male patient
D.   early loss of parent
E.   'personality deviation'

Physical Treatments

1. Current indications for electroconvulsive therapy (ECT) include

A. paranoid schizophrenia
B. puerperal depressive disorders
C. mania
D. schizodepressive psychosis
E. catatonic schizophrenia

2. Side-effects of ECT definitely include

A. mania
B. permanent long-term memory loss
C. fat embolism
D. brain damage
E. vertigo

3. Contraindications to ECT include

A. patients taking reserpine
B. coronary thrombosis in previous 5 years
C. epilepsy
D. cerebral tumour
E. raised intracranial pressure

4. Favourable features for depressive illness to respond to ECT include

A. hysterical features
B. somatic delusions
C. hypochondriasis
D. retardation
E. emotional instability

5. Names associated with the history of ECT include

A. Moniz
B. Bini
C. Ferrier
D. Cerletti
E. Freeman

6. Current indications for psychosurgery include

A. obsessional disorders
B. mania
C. chronic anxiety neurosis
D. psychopathy
E. depressive disorders

7. Side-effects of psychosurgery include

A. gross personality change ('Frankenstein')
B. apathy
C. disinhibition
D. epilepsy
E. excessive weight loss

8. Contraindications to psychosurgery include

A. cerebrovascular disease
B. drug addiction
C. schizophrenia
D. diffuse brain damage
E. alcoholism

9. The following associations are correct

A. bifrontal subcaudate tractotomy and Ballantine
B. bimedial lesions and Knight
C. orbital undercutting and Scoville
D. subcaudate lesions and Lewin
E. cingulotomies and Bridges

10. Side-effects less marked with unilateral ECT than with bilateral ECT include

A. retrograde amnesia
B. crush fractures of the vertebrae
C. nausea
D. dislocation
E. headache

Psychotherapy/Behaviour Therapy

1. **Terms associated with Adler include**

A. libido theory
B. organ superiority
C. drive for inferiority
D. fictive goals
E. psychic compensation

2. **Terms associated with Jung include**

A. ego psychology
B. analytical psychology
C. individual psychology
D. anima
E. persona

3. **Neo-freudians include**

A. Sullivan
B. Fromm
C. Horney
D. Moreno
E. Maslow

4. **Post-freudians include**

A. Wilhelm Reich
B. Otto Rank
C. Ellis
D. Erikson
E. Bowlby

5. **Terms associated with Melanie Klein include**

A. 'consensual evaluation'
B. 'object-relations'
C. play analysis
D. collective unconscious
E. paranoid position

6.   Coping behaviour in crisis intervention includes

A.   suppression
B.   regression
C.   denial
D.   sublimation
E.   inertia

7.   Problem groups in crisis intervention include

A.   conflict problems
B.   loss problems
C.   financial problems
D.   role changes
E.   problems in relationships

8.   Therapeutic factors in small group psychotherapy include

A.   intrapersonal learning
B.   shaping
C.   neurasthenia
D.   altruism
E.   universality

9.   Terms associated with Berne include

A.   structural analysis
B.   transactional analysis
C.   game analysis
D.   script analysis
E.   psychoanalysis

10.   Terms associated with Rogers include

A.   conditional positive regard
B.   paradoxical intention
C.   'basic encounters'
D.   falseness
E.   T groups

11. Features of Gestalt therapy include

A. 'marathon' groups
B. associated with Frankl
C. personification of body parts
D. associated with Perls
E. variation of sensitivity groups

12. The following associations are correct

A. Maslow and psychodrama
B. Assagioli and primal therapy
C. Frankl and existential logotherapy
D. Janov and psychosynthesis
E. Moreno and self-actualization

13. Dream work consists of

A. primary elaboration
B. displacement
C. systemization
D. dramatization
E. condensation

14. Associated mental states in paranoia characteristically include

A. turning on the self
B. magic undoing
C. reaction formation
D. splitting
E. displacement of affect

15. Concepts associated with Wilhelm Reich include

A. body armour
B. depressive position
C. orgone energy accumulator
D. neurosis originates in birth trauma
E. neurosis is due to sexual frustration

16. **Names associated with therapeutic communities include**

A. Yalom
B. Bion
C. Main
D. Maxwell-Jones
E. Ezriel

17. **Names associated with object relations theory include**

A. Freud
B. Guntrip
C. Fairbairn
D. Horney
E. Winnicot

18. **Behaviour therapy for phobias includes**

A. programmed practice
B. implosion
C. covert sensitization
D. desensitization
E. flooding treatment

19. **Behaviour therapy for general anxiety states includes**

A. progressive relaxation
B. anxiolytic drugs
C. systematic desensitization
D. insight-orientated psychotherapy
E. anxiety management training

20. **Behaviour therapy for obsessional neurosis includes**

A. social skills training
B. modelling
C. thought stopping
D. assertive training
E. response prevention

21.   Behaviour therapy for sexual deviancy includes

A.   overt sensitization
B.   continuous narcosis
C.   cyproterone acetate
D.   covert sensitization
E.   aversion therapy

22.   Cognitive distortions in depression include

A.   maladaptive assumptions
B.   undergeneralization
C.   selective abstraction
D.   positive interpretations of events
E.   arbitrary inference

23.   Self-control treatment in behaviour therapy includes

A.   self-preservation
B.   self-evaluation
C.   self-reinforcement
D.   self-monitoring
E.   self-deception

24.   The following associations are correct

A.   sexual inadequacy and 'couple therapy'
B.   enuresis and contingency management
C.   mental subnormality and 'behaviour modification'
D.   chronic schizophrenia and 'pad and bell' method
E.   marital problems and Masters and Johnson techniques

25.   Names associated with analytic group therapy include

A.   Foulkes
B.   Ferenczi
C.   Ezriel
D.   Ackerman
E.   Haley

Rehabilitation/Psychiatric Services

1.   Features of institutionalization include

A.   pauperism
B.   derealization
C.   social overstimulation
D.   loss of skills
E.   authoritarianism

2.   Historically correct dates include

A.   Bethlem Hospital, founded in 1247
B.   Guy's Hospital (lunatic ward), founded in 1728
C.   St Luke's Hospital, founded in 1751
D.   Retreat at York, founded in 1792
E.   Maudsley Hospital, opened in 1923

3.   The following acts are correctly dated

A.   Lunacy Act of 1744
B.   Vagrancy Act of 1890
C.   Mental Health (Amendment) Act of 1930
D.   Mental Treatment Act of 1982
E.   Criminal Procedure (Insanity) Act of 1964

4.   Factors associated with 'new long stay' psychiatric patients include

A.   married
B.   multiple impairments
C.   many friends or relatives
D.   good self-confidence
E.   chronic psychotic symptoms and physical disabilities

5.   Rehabilitation specifically assesses

A.   occupational skills
B.   domestic skills
C.   social skills
D.   personal attitudes
E.   behavioural analysis

Child Psychiatry

1. **Classification of child psychiatry disorders in ICD 9 includes**

A. adjustment disorder
B. attention deficit disorder
C. conduct disorder
D. hyperkinetic syndrome of childhood
E. adjustment reaction

2. **Classification of child psychiatric disorders in DSM III includes**

A. pervasive developmental disorder
B. specific delays in development
C. disturbance of conduct not elsewhere classified
D. anxiety disorders of childhood
E. specific developmental disorders

3. **Epidemiology of child psychiatric disorders includes**

A. more common in girls
B. strong correlation with social classes II and III
C. prevalence increases as intelligence increases
D. strong association with organic brain damage
E. strong association between reading retardation and conduct
    disorder

4. **Features of the WHO multi-axial classification include**

A. psychosocial problems
B. personality disorders
C. specific delays in development
D. highest level of adaptive functioning
E. intellectual level

5. **Features of short-term maternal separation (Rutter) include**

A. detatchment
B. 'deprivation dwarfism'
C. despair
D. 'affectionless psychopathy'
E. antisocial behaviour

6. **Personality tests used in children include**

A. Stanford – Binet Personality Scale
B. Rotter Sentence Completion
C. Junior Eysenck Personality Inventory
D. Gunzburg Progress Assessment Charts
E. Neale Analysis of Personality Difficulty

7. **Problems of pre-school children include**

A. pica
B. night terrors
C. attention-seeking behaviour
D. temper tantrums
E. feeding problems

8. **Epidemiology of childhood neurotic disorders includes**

A. most frequent childhood psychiatric disorders
B. obsessional disorders are the most common in mid-childhood
C. depressive disorders are commoner in younger children than in adolescence
D. hysterical disorders are frequent in adolescence
E. higher prevalence in girls

9. **Compared with the truants, the school-refusers**

A. are less depressed
B. have worse records of school work
C. are passive
D. come from less neurotic families
E. are overprotected

10. **Causes of school refusal include**

A. general social withdrawal
B. separation anxiety
C. emotional disturbance in parent
D. fear of travel
E. domestic reasons

11.   Conduct disorders include

A.   school refusal
B.   suicide
C.   juvenile delinquency
D.   truancy
E.   promiscuity

12.   ICD 9 subdivisions of conduct disorders include

A.   socialized
B.   unsocialized
C.   underinhibited
D.   non-aggressive
E.   aggressive

13.   Clinical features of the hyperkinetic syndrome include

A.   prominent antisocial behaviours
B.   temper tantrums rarely
C.   learning difficulties
D.   depression
E.   prolonged motor activity

14.   Associations of the hyperkinetic syndrome include

A.   high self-esteem
B.   'soft' neurological signs
C.   bullying
D.   epilepsy
E.   high frustration threshold

15.   Treatment of the hyperkinetic syndrome includes

A.   remedial education
B.   amphetamines
C.   methylphenidate
D.   benzodiazepines
E.   phenobarbitone

16.   Clinical features of infantile autism include

A.   loosening of associations
B.   onset before 20 months of age
C.   hallucinations
D.   obsessive desire for sameness
E.   delusions

17.   Associated features of infantile autism include

A.   stereotypies
B.   hypokinesis
C.   reduced IQ
D.   unpredictable fears
E.   self-destructive behaviour

18.   Features of 'autistic psychopathy' include

A.   begins in second year of life
B.   poor visuo-spatial perception
C.   'obsessive' preoccupations with routine
D.   poor social prognosis
E.   also called Asperger's syndrome

19.   Features of disintegrative psychoses (ICD 9) include

A.   loss of speech
B.   invariable overactivity
C.   corresponding category in DSM III
D.   invariable intellectual impairment
E.   dementia

20.   Features of specific reading retardation include

A.   writing and spelling not impaired
B.   more common in girls
C.   minor neurological abnormalities
D.   decreased prevalence in epileptic children
E.   poor attention and concentration

21. Features of specific arithmetic disorders include

A. secondary emotional difficulties
B. explained in terms of generally low IQ
C. treatment is by remedial teaching
D. prognosis is not known
E. second most common specific learning disorder

22. Causes of speech delay include

A. infantile autism
B. mental retardation
C. cerebral palsy
D. social deprivation
E. deafness

23. Epidemiology of enuresis includes

A. increased incidence in social classes I and II
B. daytime enuresis is more common in boys
C. decreased incidence in relatives
D. nocturnal enuresis is more common in girls
E. daytime enuresis has a higher prevalence than nocturnal enuresis

24. Features of enuresis include

A. nocturnal enuresis occurs after age 4
B. may be due to convulsions
C. associated with functional encopresis
D. may be due to diabetes
E. no evidence for a genetic basis

25. Emotional causes of encopresis include

A. faecal impaction with overflow incontinence
B. 'aggressive' soiling
C. Hirschsprung's disease
D. 'regressive' soiling
E. 'suppressive' soiling

26.   **Clinical features of child abuse include**

A.   rarely denied by parents
B.   retinal haemorrhage
C.   'frozen watchfulness'
D.   subdural haematoma
E.   rehydration

27.   **Factors in parents associated with child abuse include**

A.   criminal record
B.   psychiatric disorder
C.   high social class
D.   abnormal personality
E.   low rate of illegitimacy

28.   **Characteristic features of suicidal children include**

A.   usually impulsive suicidal act
B.   below-average intelligence
C.   Schaffer distinguished three groups of children
D.   apparently depressed mental state
E.   prone to violence

29.   **Differential diagnosis of tics usually includes**

A.   dyskinesias
B.   akathisia
C.   spasmodic torticollis
D.   pseudo-parkinsonism
E.   hemiballismic movements

30.   **Features of stammering include**

A.   a different disorder to stuttering
B.   more common in girls
C.   usually associated with psychiatric disorder
D.   may be treated with haloperidol
E.   usual treatment is speech therapy

Mental Handicap

1. **Synonyms of mild mental retardation (ICD 9) include**

A. moron
B. imbecile
C. highgrade defect
D. idiocy
E. feeble-minded

2. **Characteristic features of schizophrenia in mental handicap include**

A. elaborate delusions
B. poverty of thinking
C. stereotypies
D. perplexity
E. well-formed hallucinations

3. **Characteristic features of depression in mental handicap include**

A. agitation
B. retardation
C. expression of depressive ideas
D. subjective complaint of mood changes
E. compulsive behaviour

4. **Characteristic features of mania in mental handicap include**

A. pressure of speech
B. flight of ideas
C. grandoise delusions
D. episodic excitation
E. overactivity

5. **Features of epilepsy in mental handicap include**

A. associated with infantile spasms
B. common when retardation due to chromosomal abnormalities
C. uncommon when retardation due to cerebral damage
D. becomes more prevalent with increasing age
E. associated with Lennox – Gastaut syndrome

6. Causes of severe mental impairment (Mental Health Act, 1983) include

A. 15% due to Down's syndrome
B. 10% due to perinatal injury
C. 9% due to infections
D. 8% due to inherited biochemical errors
E. 50% undiagnosable

7. Features of Down's syndrome include

A. low-arched palate
B. double transverse palmar crease
C. hypertonia
D. epicanthic nasal folds
E. brushfield spots on retina

8. Down's syndrome is associated with increased incidence of

A. duodenal obstruction
B. impaired hearing
C. lymphocytic thyroiditis
D. blepharitis
E. Alzheimer's disease

9. Features of cri-du-chat syndrome include

A. deletion of short arm of chromosome 4
B. failure to thrive
C. not compatible with adult life
D. hypertelorism
E. spasticity

10. Features of phenylketonuria include

A. tyrosine hydroxylase deficiency
B. brown eyes
C. black hair
D. diagnosed prenatally by amniotic fluid culture
E. eczema

11. **Features of Tay–Sachs disease include**

A. occurs especially in Safardi Jews
B. cherry red spot on macula
C. detected prenatally with amniocentesis
D. flaccid paralysis
E. sphingomyelinase deficiency

12. **Features of Hurler's syndrome include**

A. slower deterioration than Hunter's syndrome
B. absence of corneal clouding
C. hepatosplenomegaly
D. death after adolescence
E. associated cardiac abnormalities

13. **Features of Lesch–Nyhan syndrome include**

A. post-natal diagnosis on enzyme of single hair root
B. abnormal at birth
C. scissoring position of legs
D. enzyme defect affecting pyrimidine metabolism
E. choreo-athetoid movements

14. **Features of neurofibromatosis include**

A. synonymous with epiloia
B. vitiligo
C. retardation in a minority only
D. café-au-lait spots
E. synonymous with von Münchausen syndrome

15. **Features of tuberous sclerosis include**

A. adenoma sebaceum
B. shagreen patches
C. café-au-lait spots
D. white skin patches
E. retinal phakoma

16.   Features of Lawrence – Moon – Biedl syndrome include

A.   retinitis pigmentosa
B.   polydactyly
C.   hypogenitalism
D.   obesity
E.   usually severe retardation

17.   Autosomal recessive inborn errors of metabolism include

A.   Hurler's syndrome
B.   Hunter's syndrome
C.   nephrogenic diabetes insipidus
D.   Hartnup disease
E.   Lesch – Nyhan syndrome

18.   The following associations are correct

A.   Trisomy 13 – 15 and Edwards' syndrome
B.   Trisomy 17 – 18 and Patau's syndrome
C.   XYY and Klinefelter's syndrome
D.   XO and 'fragile X' syndrome
E.   deletion of short arm of chromosome 4 and Wolf's syndrome

19.   Features of Renpenning's syndrome include

A.   abnormal ears
B.   Y-linked disorder
C.   Menkes' 'kinky hair'
D.   short stature
E.   mild handicap

20.   The phakomatoses include

A.   Sturge – Weber syndrome
B.   tuberous sclerosis
C.   Wilson's disease
D.   von Recklinghausen's disease
E.   von Hippel – Lindau disease

21.   Differential diagnosis of mental handicap usually includes

A.   affective disorder
B.   delayed maturation
C.   deafness
D.   schizophrenia
E.   personality disorder

22.   Amniocentesis may detect

A.   Gaucher's disease
B.   infantile hyperuricaemia
C.   galactosaemia
D.   maple syrup disease
E.   Lesch – Nyhan syndrome

23.   Autosomal dominant conditions include

A.   Louis – Bar syndrome
B.   Marinesco – Sjögren syndrome
C.   craniofacial dysostosis
D.   Virchow – Seckel dwarf
E.   Apert's syndrome

24.   X-linked disorders include

A.   hyperammonia syndrome
B.   Albright's syndrome
C.   Refsum's disease
D.   Lowe's syndrome
E.   Berry – Franceschetti syndrome

25.   Features of homocystinuria include

A.   dark hair and skin
B.   mild retardation
C.   ectopia lentis
D.   iridonesis
E.   malar flush

Forensic Psychiatry

1. **Testamentary capacity involves**

A. knowing the Old Testament
B. expression of oneself without ambiguity
C. the person can never be deluded
D. knowing the names of close relatives
E. being fit to drive

2. **Torts include**

A. nuisance
B. shoplifting
C. negligence
D. arson
E. trespass

3. **Correct associations in the historical development of psychopathy include**

A. Lewis and 'a most elusive category'
B. Rush and psychopathic traits
C. Kraeplin and moral derangement
D. Partridge and psychopathy
E. Henderson and sociopath

4. **The following statements about crime are definitely correct**

A. most criminals are of markedly low intelligence
B. crime in general is common among the elderly
C. crime is more common among epileptics than non-epileptics
D. depression may be associated with shop-lifting
E. homicidal threats in schizophrenics should be taken lightly

5. **Fitness to plead involves being able to**

A. examine a witness
B. understand the significance of the plea
C. instruct counsel
D. follow the progress of the trial
E. challenge a juror

6.   The various categories of _mens rea_ include

A.   blameless inadvertence
B.   _actus reus_
C.   recklessness
D.   negligence
E.   intent

7.   The McNaughton rules

A.   are named after a wood turner from Dundee
B.   have a statutory basis
C.   embody the concept of 'special verdict'
D.   can only be used if the charge is murder
E.   were drawn up at the request of the House of Lords

8.   Successful pleas in diminished responsiblity include

A.   premenstrual tension
B.   'reactive depressed state'
C.   'emotional immaturity'
D.   'mental instability'
E.   'psychopathic personality'

9.   Diminished responsibility

A.   can only be used if the charge is manslaughter
B.   refers to mental state at the time of trial
C.   is synonymous with not guilty by reason of insanity
D.   could include extreme intoxication
E.   could include 'mixed emotions of depression, disappointment and exasperation'

10.   Acts of violence committed as automatisms occur in

A.   sleep walking
B.   epileptic seizures
C.   car mechanics
D.   hypoglycaemia
E.   concussion

11. **Crimes for which 'specific intent' is required include**

A. common assault
B. manslaughter
C. indecent assault
D. rape
E. assault occasioning actual bodily harm

12. **Crimes for which 'specific intent' is not required include**

A. theft
B. arson
C. burglary
D. murder
E. assault with intent to cause grevious bodily harm

13. **Homicide is 'abnormal' if there is a finding of**

A. infanticide
B. common law manslaughter
C. diminished responsibility
D. murder
E. suicide murder

14. **Features of 'abnormal' homicide include**

A. usually committed by young men
B. homicide in women is invariably 'abnormal'
C. victims are usually family members
D. commonest psychiatric diagnosis is personality disorder
E. the commonest category in women is infanticide

15. **Classification of child murder (Scott) includes categories of**

A. infanticide
B. killing as end result of neglect
C. psychotic murder
D. mercy killing
E. suicide

16.   Recognised types of child stealing (D'Orban) include

A.   impulsive stealing in psychiatrically disturbed women
B.   manipulation with intention of influencing someone else
C.   comforting
D.   stealing for sexual gratification
E.   stealing for excitement derived from risks involved

17.   The following are offences in themselves

A.   transexualism
B.   transvestism
C.   exhibitionism
D.   'indecent exposure'
E.   'breach of the peace'

18.   Epidemiology of rape includes

A.   decreased incidence in summer
B.   70% of victims are neighbours or acquaintances
C.   increased incidence in second half of night
D.   most rapists are not mentally disordered
E.   20% of victims have a criminal record

19.   Features of indecent exposure include

A.   exhibitionism is the most frequent form
B.   may occur as an insulting gesture
C.   usually a history of psychiatric disorder
D.   reconviction rate is high
E.   many offenders proceed to more serious offences

20.   Fisher (1984) classified shoplifters into

A.   elderly shoplifters
B.   reactive shoplifters
C.   chronically bored shoplifters
D.   professional shoplifters
E.   shoplifters with severe psychiatric disorder

21. **Current epidemiology of shoplifting includes**

A. 5% incidence of psychiatric disorder
B. 5% of all shoppers shoplift at each shop
C. more common in female shoplifters
D. 'accepted perk' of shopping for some customers
E. more common in elderly shoplifters

22. **Recognised groups of arsonists include**

A. pyromaniacs
B. hypsomaniacs
C. juvenile arsonists
D. motivated arsonists
E. pathological arsonists

23. **Factors predicting that an arsonist will re-offend include**

A. no history of previous arson
B. no associated pleasure or sexual excitement
C. antisocial personality disorder
D. mental retardation
E. persistent social isolation

24. **Factors associated with dangerousness include**

A. previous willingness to delay gratification
B. paranoid traits
C. bizarre violence
D. no previous episodes of violence
E. provocation of the offence

25. **Other factors associated with dangerousness include**

A. morbid jealousy
B. continuing major denial
C. regret for the offence
D. deceptiveness
E. self control

Answers

(True responses listed)

Personality Disorder		Neurosis		Affective Disorders	
1.	C D	1.	A B C	1.	A B C D
2.	A D E	2.	A D E	2.	A B C D E
3.	C D E	3.	B C D	3.	B C D E
4.	B E	4.	A C D E	4.	C E
5.	A B D	5.	A B C D E	5.	B E
6.	A B D E	6.	A E	6.	B D E
7.	C E	7.	C E	7.	A D E
8.	A C D E	8.	B C D E	8.	D E
9.	E	9.	A B C D E	9.	B
10.	all false	10.	A B C E	10.	all false
11.	D E	11.	B C D	11.	B C
12.	A B C D E	12.	B C	12.	all false
13.	C D E	13.	E	13.	C
14.	D E	14.	all false	14.	A C E
15.	A B C D	15.	all false	15.	A C D E
16.	A B C D E	16.	A C D E	16.	A B C E
17.	B D E	17.	D	17.	E
18.	all false	18.	C E	18.	A C
19.	A B C D E	19.	E	19.	C D
20.	A B C D	20.	B D	20.	C E
		21,	A B C	21.	A C E
		22.	D E	22.	C
		23.	C E	23.	A
		24.	A B C	24.	B E
		25.	A B C D E	25.	A C E
		26.	B E	26.	A B C D E
		27.	B C D	27.	B C
		28.	A E	28.	A C D
		29.	B D E	29.	D E
		30.	D	30.	B D E

Schizophrenia

1. A C
2. B C D
3. A B D
4. A B D E
5. C D E
6. E
7. all false
8. D
9. B C E
10. A C
11. D E
12. C D
13. A B C E
14. C D E
15. B C
16. A B C D E
17. B C D
18. A C E
19. E
20. all false
21. C
22. A B D E
23. C D
24. C D E
25. A B C D E
26. A D E
27. A B D E
28. E
29. B C D E
30. C D

Paranoid Symptoms/States

1. A B C D E
2. C E
3. A E
4. C E
5. A
6. A C E
7. A B
8. A B C D E
9. C D E
10. C D
11. D E
12. all false
13. A B C D
14. B C D
15. A C D E
16. E
17. all false
18. A C E
19. A D E
20. B C E

Organic Psychiatry

1. all false
2. A E
3. A B C
4. A C E
5. A B
6. C D E
7. B D
8. D
9. C
10. A B C E
11. A B C D
12. C D
13. A B C D E
14. B C
15. A B D E
16. B C D
17. B D E
18. E
19. A
20. D E
21. B C D
22. A B C E
23. D E
24. all false
25. A B C D E
26. C D E
27. C D E
28. C E
29. A B
30. E

Psychiatry and Medicine		**Suicide/Deliberate Self-harm**		**Alcohol/Drug Dependence**	
1.	B C D	1.	all false	1.	A C D
2.	all false	2.	A C E	2.	A B C D E
3.	A B C	3.	D E	3.	C D E
4.	D E	4.	all false	4.	C D E
5.	A C D E	5.	A B C D E	5.	A E
6.	A B C D E	6.	C E	6.	A
7.	A D	7.	E	7.	all false
8.	all false	8.	B C D E	8.	A B C D E
9.	E	9.	D E	9.	E
10.	A B C D E	10.	A B C D E	10.	B C D E
11.	E	11.	B	11.	B D E
12.	A B C D	12.	C D E	12.	A C E
13.	D E	13.	A C E	13.	A E
14.	C D E	14.	A B D E	14.	A E
15.	D E	15.	B E	15.	all false
16.	A B	16.	A B C D E	16.	B E
17.	D E	17.	C	17.	A E
18.	B D E	18.	E	18.	B E
19.	B D E	19.	C D E	19.	C D E
20.	B C D E	20.	A B D E	20.	A B D E
21.	D E			21.	C E
22.	C D			22.	A C D E
23.	C			23.	D
24.	A B D E			24.	B D
25.	A C D E			25.	A B E
26.	A C E			26.	C D E
27.	B			27.	A B C
28.	D E			28.	B C D E
29.	B C E			29.	D
30.	A D E			30.	D E

Psychosexual Problems		Psychogeriatrics		Physical Treatments	
1.	B C	1.	A B C D E	1.	B D E
2.	B C	2.	all false	2.	A C E
3.	E	3.	A D	3.	A D E
4.	A B C D E	4.	C E	4.	B D
5.	A B C D E	5.	A B	5.	B D
6.	A	6.	B C E	6.	A C E
7.	C D E	7.	C D E	7.	B C D
8.	C E	8.	B E	8.	A B D E
9.	B	9.	C E	9.	C
10.	C E	10.	A B C E	10.	A C E
11.	A C D	11.	B C D E		
12.	B D	12.	all false		
13.	B D	13.	E	**Psychotherapy/**	
14.	A C E	14.	A B C D E	**Behaviour Therapy**	
15.	B D E	15.	A		
		16.	A D E	1.	D E
		17.	A B C	2.	B D E
		18.	C D	3.	A B C
		19.	E	4.	C D
		20.	A B D	5.	B C E
		21.	A B D E	6.	B C E
		22.	D E	7.	A B D E
		23.	A B D	8.	D E
		24.	B D E	9.	A B C D
		25.	A D E	10.	C E
				11.	C D
				12.	C
				13.	B D E
				14.	D
				15.	A C E
				16.	C D
				17.	B C E
				18.	A B D E
				19.	A E
				20.	B C E
				21.	D E
				22.	A C E
				23.	B C D
				24.	C
				25.	A C

Rehabilitation/ Psychiatric Services

1. A D E
2. A B C D E
3. E
4. B E
5. A B C D E

Child Psychiatry

1. D E
2. A D E
3. D E
4. A C E
5. A C
6. B C
7. A B C D E
8. all false
9. C E
10. A B D
11. D E
12. A B
13. C D E
14. B C D
15. A B C
16. D
17. A C D E
18. B C E
19. A E
20. C E
21. A C D E
22. A B C D E
23. all false
24. C
25. B D
26. B C D
27. A B D
28. D E
29. A C E
30. D E

Mental Handicap

1. A C E
2. B C D
3. A B E
4. D E
5. A E
6. all false
7. all false
8. A B C D E
9. B D E
10. E
11. B C
12. C E
13. A C E
14. B C D
15. A B C D E
16. A B C D
17. A D
18. E
19. A D
20. A B D E
21. B C
22. A B E
23. C E
24. A B D
25. C D E

Forensic Psychiatry

1. B D
2. A C E
3. A
4. D
5. A B C D E
6. A C D E
7. C E
8. A B C D E
9. D E
10. A B D E
11. all false
12. all false
13. A C E ?
14. C E
15. B C D
16. A B C
17. D E
18. D E
19. A B
20. B D E
21. A B D
22. A D E
23. C D E
24. B C
25. A B D